CARB CYCLING FOR WOMEN

A 3-Week Beginner's Step-by-Step Guide for Weight Loss With Recipes and a Meal Plan

Stephanie Hinderock

mindplusfood

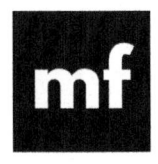

Copyright © 2020 Stephanie Hinderock

All rights reserved

No part of this book may be reproduced, or stored in a retrieval system, or transmitted in any form or by any means, electronic, mechanical, photocopying, recording, or otherwise, without express written permission of the publisher.

Printed in the United States of America0

DISCLAIMER

By reading this disclaimer, you are accepting the terms of the disclaimer in full. If you disagree with this disclaimer, please do not read the guide.

All of the content within this guide is provided for informational and educational purposes only, and should not be accepted as independent medical or other professional advice. The author is not a doctor, physician, nurse, mental health provider, or registered nutritionist/dietician. Therefore, using and reading this guide does not establish any form of a physician-patient relationship.

Always consult with a physician or another qualified health provider with any issues or questions you might have regarding any sort of medical condition. Do not ever disregard any qualified professional medical advice or delay seeking that advice because of anything you have read in this guide. The information in this guide is not intended to be any sort of medical advice and should not be used in lieu of any medical advice by a licensed and qualified medical professional.

The information in this guide has been compiled from a variety of known sources. However, the author cannot attest to or guarantee the accuracy of each source and thus should not be held liable for any errors or omissions.

You acknowledge that the publisher of this guide will not be held liable for any loss or damage of any kind incurred as a result of this guide or the reliance on any information provided within this guide. You acknowledge and agree that you assume all risk and responsibility for any action you undertake in response to the information in this guide.

Using this guide does not guarantee any particular result (e.g., weight loss or a cure). By reading this guide, you acknowledge that there are no guarantees to any specific outcome or results you can expect.

All product names, diet plans, or names used in this guide are for identification purposes only and are the property of their respective owners. The use of these names does not imply endorsement. All other trademarks cited herein are the property of their respective owners.

Where applicable, this guide is not intended to be a substitute for the original work of this diet plan and is, at most, a supplement to the original work for this diet plan and never a direct substitute. This guide is a personal expression of the facts of that diet plan.

Where applicable, persons shown in the cover images are stock photography models and the publisher has obtained the rights to use the images through license agreements with third-party stock image companies.

CONTENTS

Title Page
Copyright
Disclaimer
Introduction — 1
What Is Carb Cycling? — 3
Girl Power: Carb Cycling for Women — 10
A Potential Five-Step Guide to Getting Started — 15
Weekly Guide — 19
Delights for Carb Rights — 23
Healthy High-Carb Recipes — 24
Healthy Low-Carb Recipes — 29
Conclusion — 49
References and Helpful Links — 51

INTRODUCTION

Do you want to lose weight quickly while still enjoying the carbs you intake? If yes, you're in the right place to learn how.

If you want to lose fats by just alternating the intake of carbohydrates, then read this article until the last portion. While reading this, you will garner ideas and knowledge about Carb Cycling for Women.

By its definition, Carb Cycling is another process of reducing fats and maintaining physical fitness by altering your carb intake. It is a dietary method on a daily, weekly, or monthly basis. Moreover, Carb Cycling's main goal is to organize carbohydrate intake when it delivers an extreme advantage and remove carbohydrates when they are not needed.

Carb Cycling is ideal for bodybuilders and other high-performing athletes but it can also be used by people who want to become physically fit.

Did you know that this dietary approach seems more efficient compared to others? It is because other approaches to intensive dieting result in most dieters failing to maintain their long-term plans. Unlike Carb Cycling, it is way easier to manage your diet plan by just adjusting your carb intake. There are suggested diet plans you can follow when you are going to start your Carb

Cycling journey which you will encounter examples in the final chapter of this book.

In this guide, you will discover...
- What carb cycling is
- The background information around carb cycling
- The benefits of carb cycling as it pertains to women
- How carb cycling works
- A potential 5-step guide to getting started with carb cycling
- Weekly plans and tips
- Common and curated recipes that are tasty and fun to make

If you would like to learn more, continue reading this guide, as we go through this journey step-by-step.

WHAT IS CARB CYCLING?

Overview

Carb cycling is a popular diet plan among women who are looking to lose weight and improve their overall health. It involves increasing and decreasing the number of carbohydrates one consumes regularly, allowing for periods where carbohydrates are the focus and other times when they are taken out of the diet plan altogether. Carb cycling can be an effective way to achieve results while avoiding the dreaded "plateau" that often comes during long-term dieting.

Foods to Eat

In carb cycling, usually, there are high-carb days followed by low-carb days.

High-carb days

On high-carb days, it is important to focus on complex carbohydrates such as:

• Whole grain bread – High in complex carbohydrates to fuel your workout, whole grain bread is an excellent source of energy and fiber.

• Fruit – Fruits are packed with vitamins and minerals, as well as being full of natural sugar for a quick boost of energy. Try to choose fruits that are low in fructose, such as apples and bananas.

• Oats – Oats contain soluble fiber which helps to keep you feeling full for longer and can help moderate blood sugar levels throughout the day. They're great for a pre-workout snack or added to protein shakes.

- Brown rice – Brown rice is another complex carbohydrate that provides sustained energy throughout your workout. It's also a good source of magnesium and vitamin B6, both essential for muscle growth and recovery after exercise.

- Sweet potatoes– Sweet potatoes are high in carbs but also low on the glycemic index, making them ideal for anyone following a carb-cycling diet on high-carb days. They're also packed with vitamins A and C, as well as magnesium which can all aid muscle and tissue repair after exercise.

- Quinoa– Quinoa is high in carbohydrates and proteins and also contains iron, potassium, zinc, and vitamin B6. It's a good option to add during carb-cycling on high-carb days as it provides sustained energy throughout the day.

- Whole wheat pasta – Whole wheat pasta is an excellent complex carbohydrate when following a carb-cycling diet on high-carb days. Packed with essential vitamins and minerals like magnesium, phosphorus, folate, thiamin, niacin, riboflavin, and zinc, whole wheat pasta is an ideal source of energy for exercising.

- Legumes – Legumes are packed with protein and fiber as well as vital micronutrients. Perfect for maintaining muscle mass when following a low-carb diet on off days, legumes are also a great source of sustained energy for those on high-carb days. Try adding lentils or chickpeas to your meals for added benefits.

These will provide the body with important nutrients, vitamins, and minerals that support healthy functioning and muscle growth.

Low-carb days
On low-carb days, women should focus on lean protein sources such as:

- Eggs - This high-protein food is packed with essential amino acids and healthy fats, making it an ideal food item for low-carb days.

• Spinach - Rich in vitamins A and C, this leafy green vegetable is low in carbs and a great addition to any meal on a carb-cycling diet.

• Avocado - This superfood has healthy monounsaturated fats that are beneficial for weight loss and provide satiety on a low-carb day.

• Nuts and seeds - These crunchy snacks offer plenty of protein and high amounts of healthy fats. Opt for raw or lightly roasted nuts such as almonds, walnuts, sunflower seeds, chia seeds, etc.

• Fish - High in omega-3 fatty acids, fish is a lean source of protein that should be included regularly when following a carb-cycling diet.

• Cheese - Full of protein and calcium, cheese can help to keep you feeling full throughout the day on your low-carb days.

• Greek yogurt - Dairy products like Greek yogurt contain calcium and probiotics that can help improve digestion while also providing important nutrients to the body.

• Legumes - Beans like chickpeas, black beans, and lentils all offer plant-based proteins as well as fiber that can help regulate blood sugar levels during carbohydrate restriction.

Eating adequate amounts of protein helps to keep hunger at bay throughout the day so that you don't feel deprived or overly hungry.

Lifestyle Changes to Make Carb Cycling Work
Whether you're just starting on a carb cycling diet or looking to optimize an existing one, implementing these lifestyle changes can significantly help make managing the cycle easier.

• Get Adequate Sleep: Getting adequate sleep is essential for any fitness regimen. Not only does insufficient sleep affect our mood and ability to concentrate throughout the day, but it can also disrupt our hormones, making carb cycling more difficult to maintain. Women should aim for 7-9 hours of quality sleep per night.

- Incorporate Intermittent Fasting: Incorporating intermittent fasting into a carb-cycling diet can be beneficial for several reasons. First, it's easier to stick to a low-carb eating plan if meals are spaced out properly throughout the day. Second, intermittent fasting helps stimulate fat burning by keeping insulin levels low.

- Exercise Regularly: Exercise is an important part of any lifestyle and carb cycling is no exception. Working out regularly helps increase energy levels and burn calories more efficiently – two key elements in successful weight loss or weight management goals with carb cycling. Women should aim for 3-4 days of resistance training per week along with light cardio on non-resistance days.

- Reduce Stress: As with many diets, stress can become one of the biggest obstacles to staying on track with your eating plan. Besides taking time each day specifically devoted to relaxation activities such as meditation or yoga, reducing stress hormones (cortisol) is key in successful carb cycling as high cortisol levels lead to insulin spikes which would decrease the effectiveness of the cycle itself.

Benefits from Carb Cycling
Carb cycling can provide numerous benefits for women, such as improved cognitive function, increased metabolism, reduced body fat, improved hormone balance, more energy, boosted mood regulation, decreased inflammation, and increased nutrient absorption. Here are 8 specific benefits of carb cycling:

1. Improved Cognitive Function: Carb cycling can help improve mental sharpness and focus by regulating blood sugar levels and reducing inflammation in the body. Additionally, it can help balance hormones related to hunger, cravings, and energy

production.

2. Increased Metabolism: Regular carb cycling can boost fat-burning capabilities by manipulating insulin levels. This helps your body adjust to its optimal rate for calorie burning efficiently thus improving overall metabolism.

3. Reduced Body Fat: When you cycle carbs, you experience a reduction in stored body fat due to improved insulin sensitivity, increased calorie-burning capabilities, and increased thermogenesis (heat production).

4. Improved Hormone Balance: Intermittent fasting or carb cycling can restore normal hormonal balance in women who are struggling with imbalanced hormones such as thyroid or cortisol-related issues.

5. More Energy: When done correctly carb cycling will provide sustained energy throughout the day without the crash and burn often associated with yo-yo dieting or other unhealthy eating styles that rely on quick fixes of processed carbohydrates or sugary snacks.

6. Boosted Mood Regulation: One benefit of carb cycling is its ability to regulate serotonin levels which play an essential role in both mood regulation and appetite control—two factors that are very important for women's overall health and well-being!

7. Decreased Inflammation: Cycling carbs has been shown to reduce inflammation throughout the body caused by poor dietary choices—this can mean decreased risk for chronic diseases like diabetes and heart disease as well as improved joint health!

8. Increased Nutrient Absorption: Lastly, when done correctly, carb cycling will help your body absorb essential vitamins & minerals from your food more effectively - this means higher levels of nutrients needed for optimal health!

By following a carb cycling plan, women can experience

numerous physical and mental health benefits that can last beyond the initial dieting phase.

Overall, carb cycling can be an effective way for women to lose weight while enjoying some indulgences along the way; it also offers flexibility which makes it easier to stick with it long term. Note that this type of diet may not work for everyone due to individual lifestyle needs; always consult your physician before starting any new regimen and listen closely to what your body tells you when making dietary changes.

Is Carb Cycling safe?
Carb cycling is an effective approach for women to manage their diets because it enables them to lose or maintain weight while still enjoying the benefits of having carbs in their meals. Carb cycling allows women to enjoy the benefits of having carbs in their meals while still losing or maintaining weight. It can assist women in obtaining the necessary nutrients and maintaining an active lifestyle. Carb cycling, when performed properly, can assist you in reaching your fitness objectives without putting your health in jeopardy.

Alternating between days with a high carbohydrate intake and days with a reduced carbohydrate intake is how this method works. When following a low-carb diet, the majority of one's daily calorie intake should come from protein and fat, with just a little amount of room left over for carbs. When you consume a diet heavy in carbs, you should aim to get between 50 and 65 percent of your daily calories from nutritious carbohydrates like oatmeal, sweet potatoes, legumes, quinoa, fruits, and whole grains.

When opposed to the practice of constantly consuming simple sweets, this technique helps manage blood sugar levels; in addition to supplying satiation and energy throughout the day, it also offers sufficient fuel for physical activity. Consuming fewer carbohydrates on certain days paves the way for you to have a greater quantity of carbs on other days without going over your daily calorie limit.

Because of this, it is much easier to stick to the diet because you don't have to exclude any food categories! In addition, consuming a suitable amount of protein and fats will help control appetite and supply crucial nutrients for either increasing muscle mass or decreasing body fat, depending on the fitness objective you have set for yourself.

Carb cycling is not for everyone; its principles should be adapted according to an individual's activity level and biochemistry; nonetheless, if it is done correctly, it may be a safe alternative for women who are trying to manage their diets.

The most important thing you can do is make sure that the majority of your carbohydrates come from whole foods rather than processed "junk" foods. This is because whole foods contain the highest concentration of micronutrients and pose the lowest risk of disrupting digestion or raising blood glucose levels.

Before you get started with carb cycling, it is a good idea to consult with a nutritionist who is knowledgeable about the practice. This will allow you to create a personalized diet that is rational and appropriate for your circumstances.

GIRL POWER: CARB CYCLING FOR WOMEN

These days, especially for women, body health, is one of the factors that plays a very important role in this fast pace time of life, which is why some people stick with a wide variety of internet diets and exercise for two main different reasons; to lessen the gym training duration or maximize the gym training efforts

Aside from the keto diet, it's been introduced already that the process of carb cycling is quite popular nowadays, especially for people in training for strength sports.

Many research articles are explaining the benefits and principles of this diet by commonly considering men under this diet as an example. The question is could women have the accessibility to gain the benefits of carb cycling also? The answer is an absolute yes. They can have a greater tendency to accumulate unnecessary fat tissues than men.

The Advantages of Carb Cycling for Women
So if you're a kind of woman looking for a new kind of diet routine, here are the reasons why you should pick carb cycling:

It's not that overly complicated.
Carb cycling is a kind of flexible dieting approach thus it doesn't

have any complicated rules. All you need is to follow your weekly routine but in a restrictive and limited way, take note that rules apply and intake guidelines still count if you want to see them.

Boosts work efficiency for the whole day, especially in workouts.
Having more consumption of carbohydrates during intense workouts or even physical activities results in muscle glycogen being stored which will be converted into glucose for the body that is more efficient in much more intense and longer workouts or other physical activities which reflects the increase in work efficiency.

A good pick for muscle gain objectives.
If you want to gain some muscles, a caloric surplus is a must. On the other hand, women under workout or training days must eat 200 to 300 calories above their maintenance and keep these calories around their maintenance during off-training days.

Maintaining this lessens or even blocks the possibility of fat gain allowing you to recover from heavy training. Besides, if carb cycling is added and maintained, it increases the heavy workout time duration for your muscle gain.

More carbs, less water retention for the body.
Having many carbs in your body especially, results in retaining the water in the body, especially during low physical activities and even before your menstrual cycle visits. Overall, carb cycling reduces this kind of phenomenon to a minimum level.

It ups the cells' sensitivity to glucose.
When having a low carb intake, improves insulin sensitivity, especially glucose which is very important for gaining body shape.

Some women share their stories within the "before and after changes" in their carb cycling which is a big factor in how carb cycling is quite effective for improving body composition. Here are the stories being shared on social platforms about their carb-cycling journey.

One of the success stories of carb cycling is the story of Nicole Collet. Based on her story, her partner used to work out five times a week, following the guidelines of intake for carbohydrates, fats, and protein. "The carbs specifically defueled the muscles," she said in support of her statement that they focused on taking carbs for workout training. With this, the result is as Collet loses a hundred pounds of fat in her.

Lastly, don't forget to track your progress over time with food logs or fitness apps—this can help you review how certain cycles have impacted your body composition goals while also helping you ascertain what cycle works best for you.

Women Who Could Benefit from Carb Cycling
Women who are looking to reach their fitness and health goals can benefit from the carb-cycling diet. This type of diet plan allows them to reap the benefits of increasing and decreasing carbohydrate consumption to maintain progress while controlling their cravings.

• Active Women: Busy women who live an active lifestyle, such as working professionals and gym-goers, will benefit greatly from carb cycling. It helps them maintain energy levels so that they can stay consistent with their exercise routines and avoid plateaus in their progress.

• Absentee Dieters: Women who have trouble staying consistent with a set diet will find it easier to stick with carb cycling since it involves alternating the number of carbs consumed on certain days rather than completely cutting out carbs indefinitely.

• Competitive Athletes: Carb cycling is ideal for competitive athletes because it maximizes fat loss without compromising muscle or performance-enhancing nutrients like carbohydrates. By controlling how many carbs you consume, your body is better able to regulate its energy levels without sacrificing strength or endurance during competition.

- Health Conscious Women: All women should be conscious about what they eat to stay healthy, but carb cycling offers an opportunity for those who want to focus on healthy eating while still enjoying the occasional cheat meal or snack. By monitoring carb intake, women can make sure they stay on track while still indulging once in a while guilt-free!

- Weight Loss Seekers: Carb cycling is a great way for women to control their portions and regulate their caloric intake without feeling deprived or overly restricted. This type of diet allows them to enjoy the occasional splurge while still maintaining healthy habits. In addition, carb cycling can help speed up weight loss by burning off excess fat instead of muscle when calories are decreased.

- Stress Eaters: Stress eating is a common problem for many women, and carb cycling can be used to help combat cravings triggered by emotional eating. When done correctly, this type of diet helps reduce stress hormones like cortisol so that the body no longer relies on carbohydrates as a source of comfort or reward.

No matter your health and fitness goals, carb cycling can be an effective tool to help women stay on track.

Who Should NOT Follow The Carb Cycling Diet?
Carb cycling has some potential health benefits, but certain women should avoid the diet due to existing medical conditions or the risk of developing unhealthy eating habits.

- Women with Diabetes: Carb cycling is not recommended for women with diabetes, since it can be difficult to predict how the changes in carbohydrate intake will affect insulin levels.

- Women who are pregnant: Pregnant women should not follow a carb-cycling diet because their bodies need more calories and nutrients and there is no evidence that carb cycling has any added benefit during pregnancy.

- Women with adrenal fatigue: Carb cycling may worsen symptoms of existing adrenal fatigue because the sporadic fluctuations in blood sugar can create further stress on an already-taxed endocrine system.

- Women with thyroid disorders: The fluctuations in blood sugar associated with a carb-cycling diet can adversely affect the functioning of the thyroid gland, making it difficult to manage symptoms of an underlying disorder.

- Women with gastrointestinal issues: Carb cycling can be problematic for women with gastrointestinal issues as it may exacerbate existing symptoms such as bloating, constipation, and/or diarrhea.

- Women with eating disorders: Carb cycling can be particularly dangerous in individuals prone to disordered eating behavior because it could trigger an unhealthy obsession with food and macronutrient ratios.

- Women recovering from illness or surgery: Individuals who have recently experienced a major illness or surgery should not follow a carb-cycling diet since sudden shifts in nutrition can impede healing and recovery.

In general, carb cycling should be considered with caution, especially for the women mentioned above.

A POTENTIAL FIVE-STEP GUIDE TO GETTING STARTED

Carb cycling is a diet plan which involves alternating between high- and low-carb days to keep your body in an optimal nutrient balance. This can help you reach your health and fitness goals, whether they include weight loss, muscle building, or fat burning. In this guide, we'll take you through the five steps to get started with carb cycling and make sure that it's the right diet for you.

Step 1. Familiarize yourself with the basics of Carb Cycling
Before you get started, it's important to understand how carb cycling works and why it can be beneficial for your body. Carb cycling involves alternating between days of high-carb consumption and low-carb consumption, to keep your body in an optimal nutrient balance. During the high-carb days, you'll consume more carbs than you would normally, allowing for increased energy levels for workouts and fat burning on subsequent low-carb days. Additionally, high-carb diets can lead to a general feeling of well-being because they are known to increase serotonin levels—hormones that regulate mood.

Meanwhile, lowering carb intake on days when you're not as active works towards enabling fat burning. It's also helpful to know some of the caveats associated with carb cycling before starting this diet plan. First, it requires greater effort since each day requires different macronutrients and foods; carbohydrate sources change from high- to low-carb days which means planning meals in advance is essential.

Furthermore, following a strict cycle, every week could lead to nutrient deficiency if your diet lacks variety or doesn't provide sufficient micro and macronutrients for optimal health. Therefore, it's recommended that you follow a balanced diet even during your periods of high/low carbs intake so that any micronutrient deficiencies are avoided. By understanding these basics of the carb cycling lifestyle you will have the tools necessary to make informed decisions about what's best for your body as you start on this journey!

Step 2. Assess your goals and current health and fitness levels
Starting your carb cycling lifestyle requires you to assess your goals and current health and fitness levels. It's essential to understand what you hope to achieve with this diet plan as this will influence the structure of your cycle.

If your end goal is weight loss, a simple carb cycling plan might be best suited; alternate between high-carb intake days and low-carb intake days (for example, five high-carb days, followed by two low-carb days). However, if gaining muscle mass, or improving athletic performance is your main aim then a more complex approach could work better for you, for instance breaking down each week into daily nutrition for each macronutrient.

In addition to setting achievable goals, it's important to take into consideration any pre-existing health conditions or allergies that might affect how you decide upon a carb cycling pattern. Speak with your doctor or nutritionist to find out whether carb cycling is right for you based on the specifics of your situation.

Remembering that specific caloric needs vary from individual to individual is key when starting any new diet plan, so make sure that whatever carb cycle pattern you go with matches up with yours!

Step 3. Decide on a schedule and pick your foods
This involves establishing which days will be high-carb, low-carb, and no-carb days. It's important to note that you'll find the biggest benefits of carb cycling by having a consistent pattern that works for you week in and week out. When it comes to choosing which foods to consume, keep in mind that during high-carb days, you'll want to focus on complex carbs such as oats, whole wheat or rye bread, brown rice, and sweet potatoes.

These carbs provide your body with long-lasting energy which will allow you to perform well when exercising or training. Meanwhile, low-carb days focus on eating lean meats such as chicken, turkey, and salmon with non-starchy vegetables like broccoli and spinach for added vitamins and minerals. This process may take some trial and error before finding what works best for you - so don't feel discouraged if an initial cycle doesn't work out as planned!

Step 4. Pair your meals with the right workout type
Depending on your goals and the cycle you are following, there may be different recommendations for each day.

For instance, if you're in between high-carb and low-carb days and are still interested in gaining muscle mass or strength, you should opt for a heavier weight training session that targets major muscle groups while keeping rest periods short. During low-carb days, however, it's important to focus on bodyweight exercises such as HIIT workouts or yoga which require less energy but still provide an effective exercise session.

On no-carb days, it may be best to go for a recovery day to rest and re-energize—going for a relaxed walk or a light swim can make all the difference! For more experienced athletes who are looking to build endurance during their carb-cycling journey, aerobic exercises can also be included as appropriate. Remember that whatever exercise routine you decide upon should sync with your diet's caloric needs as well as specific goals. We'll provide a sample workout plan that you may follow in the following chapter.

By combining the correct diet pattern and exercise regimen - you'll find yourself well on your way to achieving optimal fitness levels with this lifestyle change!

Step 5. Supplement correctly
While diet and exercise are important, supplementation plays an equally vital role in helping you reach your fitness goals. For example, multivitamins, protein powders, and fish oil supplements can all be useful in providing extra vitamins and minerals throughout your cycle period.

Additionally, depending on your fitness goals, certain specialized supplements may need to be taken. If you're looking to build muscle mass or strength, BCAAs may help reduce fatigue while also helping with muscle recovery post-workout. On the other hand, if fat loss is your goal, adding a quality greens powder such as spirulina or wheatgrass might be beneficial for keeping hunger pangs at bay while boosting overall nutrition levels.

Be aware that it's always best to talk with a certified nutritionist or registered dietician before considering any form of supplementation—as they can better advise you on which type of supplement will suit your needs best without compromising your health status. With a little guidance from experts—supplements could become an effective part of a successful carb cycling journey!

WEEKLY GUIDE

The First Week of Carb Cycling Journey
Are you looking for a Carb Cycling diet plan? You can follow the weekly diet plan stated below. It was mentioned earlier that Carb Cycling is the process of alternating the intake of carbohydrates that's why it is necessary to have an organized plan.

In this guide, there will be a 3-week diet plan. Every week, there will be a minimal change in carbohydrate intake. Furthermore, there will be a variation of physical activities, and carb and fat intake to maintain the balance.

There are 2 common methods of Carb Cycling. These are The High/Low Method and The High/Medium/Low Method.

The High/Low Method – in this method, you will be undergoing a high-carb day followed by a low-carb day. High carb day must cover at least 150 grams of carbohydrates intake while low carb day must cover at most 100 grams of carbohydrates intake.

The High/Medium/Low Method – in this method you will be undergoing a high-carb day followed by a medium-carb day and eventually a low-carb day. High carb day must cover at least 150 grams of carbohydrates intake, medium carb day must cover between 100-150 grams of carbohydrates intake, while low carb day must cover at most 100 grams of carbohydrates intake.

Below is a diet plan table for week 1

Day	Exercise	Carb Intake	Fat Intake	Carb Amount
Monday	Weight Training	High Carb	Low Fat	200 g
Tuesday	Aerobic Exercise	Mod Carb	Mod Fat	100 g
Wednesday	Rest Day	Low Carb	High Fat	30 g
Thursday	Weight Training	High Carb	Low Fat	200 g
Friday	Weight Training	High Carb	Low Fat	200 g
Saturday	Rest Day	Low Carb	High Fat	30 g
Sunday	Rest Day	Low Carb	High Fat	30 g

Meanwhile, to make your diet plan more efficient, there are certain rules and guidelines you must consider.

In research, it was found that most people eating meals within an 8-10-hour gap burn more fatty acids, enhance insulin sensitivity, and reduce damaged cells. Thus, you must eat your meals within an exact gap.

Protein can be an essential agent to create weight loss through soothing blood sugar and sustaining muscle mass. Thus, you must eat 20-40 grams of protein during your meals.

Fiber supports the regulation of blood sugar, which is necessary to maintain regular body weight. Fiber can be gained by eating fruits and vegetables. Thus, you must eat vegetables during your meals.

Prefer whole foods rather than powdered ones. To improve body composition, you need to intake around 3-6 grams of omega 3 fatty acids during your meal.

On the other hand, there are also certain things you need to avoid during your Carb Cycling diet.

Avoid flavored beverages and drinks. This kind of drink may be a hindrance to your progress during your diet properly. It is advisable to drink water and unsweetened teas rather than flavored ones.

Follow your meal plan. Do not cheat on your plan to achieve progress within a couple of days or weeks.

Avoid sauces. It is better to use spices rather than sauces like ketchup and dressings. This kind of seasoning contains a high amount of carbohydrates.

Second Week of Carb Cycling Journey
After your first week of the Carb Cycling journey, there are still two more weeks. For the second week, here is a diet plan you can follow.

Day	Exercise	Carb Intake	Fat Intake	Carb Amount
Monday	Weight Training	High Carb	Low Fat	250 g
Tuesday	Aerobic Exercise	Mod Carb	Mod Fat	150 g
Wednesday	Rest Day	No Carb	High Fat	0 g
Thursday	Weight Training	High Carb	Low Fat	250 g
Friday	Aerobic Exercise	Mod Carb	Mod Fat	150 g
Saturday	Rest Day	Low Carb	High Fat	100 g
Sunday	Rest Day	No Carb	High Fat	0 g

As you're in two weeks of the carb cycling process, you should restrict your meal diet and keep the following tips mentioned before in the first week of the carb cycling diet.

Third Week of Carb Cycling Journey

Here you go, the third week of your carb cycle journey, the table below is an example of a simultaneous carb cycling process for the third week. However, take note that you can repeat your routine for another week depending on what's in your guts.

After the first two weeks of the Carb Cycling journey, you can continue this for more weeks based on your body's needs. For the third week, here is a diet plan you can follow.

Day	Exercise	Carb Intake	Fat Intake	Carb Amount
Monday	Weight Training	High Carb	Low Fat	250 g
Tuesday	Aerobic Exercise	Mod Carb	Mod Fat	150 g
Wednesday	Weight Training	High Carb	High Fat	250 g
Thursday	Rest Day	No Carb	Low Fat	0 g
Friday	Aerobic Exercise	Mod Carb	Mod Fat	150 g
Saturday	Rest Day	Low Carb	High Fat	100 g
Sunday	Rest Day	Low Carb	High Fat	100 g

Still, the remarks for this week's routine are to follow the tips and guides in the first-week process and see the effectiveness of Carb Cycling.

If you want to enhance your carb cycling diet, try to keep track of your carb cycling calculator or try to put your routine in a PDF file, or any schedule organizer can track and keep your carb cycling in the process.

DELIGHTS FOR CARB RIGHTS

As you finish understanding and learning what carb cycling is and the step-by-step implementation within three weeks, this chapter provides five high and low-carb recipes that you might want or need to add to your meal plan.

HEALTHY HIGH-CARB RECIPES

Carrot Cake Oats

Ingredients:
- 1/2 cup dry oats, cooked in water
- 1 scoop vanilla whey protein powder
- 3 oz. unsweetened almond milk
- 2-3 tbsp. carrots, grated
- allspice, to taste
- cinnamon, to taste
- nutmeg, to taste
- 1 tbsp. maple syrup
- Optional: 1 tbsp. sliced almonds
- Optional: 1 tbsp. shaved coconut

Instructions:
1. Prepare cooked oats in a bowl.
2. In a shaker bottle, mix almond milk and protein powder vigorously until well-mixed.
3. Add to the serving of oatmeal and mix.
4. Add the remaining ingredients. Stir well.
5. Serve as is or warm up the oatmeal in the microwave before serving.

Chicken and Broccoli Casserole

Ingredients:
- 1 tbsp. olive oil
- 1/2 red onion, diced
- 1 tbsp. garlic, minced
- 1 cup uncooked brown rice
- 1 tsp. rosemary
- 1 tsp. thyme
- 1 lb. chicken breast, chopped into 1-inch pieces
- 3-1/2 cups low sodium chicken broth
- 1/2 cup (4 oz.) 2% Greek yogurt
- 2/3 cup 3-cheese blend
- 12 oz. raw broccoli florets

Instructions:
1. Set the slow cooker to low heat sauté function
2. Sauté olive oil, garlic, and onion until the onions caramelize.
3. Add uncooked brown rice, fresh rosemary, and fresh thyme.
4. Mix well. Ensure that every grain of rice is covered in the seasoning.
5. Add in chicken broth, followed by raw chicken breasts. Stir.
6. Pop the top of the slow cooker. Adjust to medium-high heat and cook for 3 to 5 hours.
7. An hour before the cooking time ends, mix it again.
8. Put in cheese and Greek yogurt. Mix it until creamy.
9. Add florets on top of the rice.
10. Season to taste with sea salt and pepper.

Sweet Potato Salad

Ingredients:
- 3 sweet potatoes, large, peeled
- 2 celery stalks, chopped
- 1 red bell pepper, diced
- 1/2 medium red onion, diced

Sauce:
- 2 tbsp. 2% Greek yogurt
- 1 tsp. smoked paprika
- 1/4 cup safflower mayo
- 1 tbsp. Dijon mustard
- cumin, to taste
- fresh orange juice
- sea salt, to taste
- pepper, to taste
- optional: 1 tsp. fresh rosemary
- optional: pinch of turmeric

Garnish:
- fresh chopped green onion
- 1/2 cup goat cheese crumble, may adjust the amount to taste

Instructions:
1. Boil sweet potatoes until tender, about 12-15 minutes. Strain and set aside to cool down.
2. Mix together the ingredients for the sauce. Season to taste with sea salt & pepper.
3. Chop the sweet potato into chunks.
4. Transfer the sweet potato to a large bowl. Add in chopped veggies, and top with the sauce. Fold them gently together.
5. Serve warm or chilled.

Cajun-Style Chicken Wrap

Ingredients:
- 1 large whole wheat keto tortilla
- 1/2 avocado, chopped
- 4 oz. cajun chicken, breast part, chopped and cooked
- 1/2 beefsteak tomato, chopped
- 2 tbsp. yogurt, preferably plain or organic
- 1-1/2 cups lettuce, chopped
- 1/3 cup cucumber, chopped
- pepper, to taste
- sea salt, to taste

Instructions:
1. Except for the tortilla, toss all the ingredients for the salad in a bowl.
2. Heat up the tortilla in the microwave for 15 seconds, then plate it nicely.
3. Gently transfer the salad mix to the center of the tortilla. Once done, fold both sides nicely, similar to how a burrito is wrapped.
4. Slice and enjoy eating.

HEALTHY LOW-CARB RECIPES

Egg Salad with Avocados

Ingredients:
- 3 medium-sized avocados
- 6 eggs, large and hard-boiled
- 1/3 red onion, medium size
- 3 celery ribs
- 4 tbsp. mayonnaise
- 2 tbsp. freshly squeezed lime juice
- 2 tsp. brown mustard
- 1/2 tsp. cumin powder
- 1 tsp. hot sauce
- salt
- pepper

Instructions:
1. Chop the eggs, celery, and onion.
2. Set aside the avocados, then combine the rest of the ingredients.
3. Slice the avocado in half to take out the pit.
4. Stuff the avocado by spooning the egg salad on its cave.
5. Serve and enjoy.

Roasted Veggies

Ingredients:
- 1/2 lb. turnips
- 1/2 lb. carrots
- 1/2 lb. parsnips
- 2 shallots, peeled
- 1/4 tsp. ground black pepper
- 1 tbsp. extra-virgin olive oil
- 6 cloves garlic
- 3/4 tsp. kosher salt
- 2 tbsp. fresh rosemary needles

Instructions:
1. First, cut vegetables into bite-sized pieces.
2. Set the oven to 400°F.
3. Mix all the ingredients in a baking dish.
4. Roast the vegetables for 25 minutes until brown and tender.
5. Toss and roast again for 20–25 minutes.
6. Serve and enjoy while hot.

Keto Zucchini Walnut Bread

Ingredients:
- 3 large eggs
- 1/2 cup virgin olive oil
- 1 tsp. vanilla extract
- 2-1/4 cups fine almond flour
- 1-1/2 cups sweetener, erythritol
- 1/2 tsp. salt
- 1-1/2 tsp. baking powder
- 1/2 tsp. nutmeg, ground
- 1 tsp. cinnamon, ground
- 1/4 tsp. ginger, ground
- 1 cup zucchini, grated
- 1/2 cup walnuts, chopped

Instructions:
1. Preheat your oven to 350°F.
2. Whisk together the eggs, oil, and vanilla extract. Set aside.
3. Using another bowl, combine the baking powder, sweetener, almond flour, salt, cinnamon, nutmeg, and ginger powder. Set aside.
4. Squeeze the excess water from the zucchini using a paper towel or a cheesecloth.
5. Pour the zucchini into the egg mixture and whisk.
6. Add the flour mixture slowly into the egg and zucchini mixture. Blend using an electric blender until the mixture turns smooth.
7. Spray a loaf pan with avocado oil or baking spray.
8. Pour the zucchini batter into the loaf pan and smoothen the top evenly.
9. Spoon the chopped walnuts on top of the batter, lightly pressing the walnuts with the back of a spoon to press into the batter.
10. Pop the loaf pan into the oven and then bake for 60-70 minutes, or until the walnuts turn brown.
11. Cool in a cooling rack before slicing and serving.

Tangy Lemon Fish

Ingredients:
- 200 g. Gurnard fresh fish fillets
- 3 tbsp. butter
- 1 tbsp. fresh lemon juice
- 1/4 cup fine almond flour
- 1 tsp. dried dill
- 1 tsp. dried chives
- 1 tsp. onion powder
- 1/2 tsp. garlic powder
- salt
- pepper

Instructions:
1. On a large plate or tray, combine dill, almond flour, and spices. Mix until well combined.
2. Dredge each fillet one at a time into the flour mix. Turn the fillet around until fully coated, and then transfer to a clean plate or tray. This may be refrigerated until ready to cook.
3. Place a large pan over medium-high heat.
4. Combine halves of butter and lemon juice. Swirl the pan to mix, lift occasionally to avoid burning the butter.
5. Allow the fish to cook for about 3 minutes.
6. Let the fish absorb all the lemony-butter mixture. Cook on low heat to avoid drying out the pan.
7. Add the remaining lemon juice and butter to the pan.
8. Turn the fish to cook the other side for 3 minutes more. Swirl around the pan to fully coat it with the juice.
9. Wait until it turns golden brown and the fish is cooked through.
10. Serve with buttered vegetables.

Spinach and Watercress Salad

Ingredients:
- 1 cup watercress, washed with stems removed
- 3 cups baby spinach, washed with stems removed
- 1 medium sliced avocado
- 1/4 cup avocado oil
- 1/8 cup lemon juice
- a pinch of salt

Instructions:
1. Pat dry the spinach and watercress. Remove the stem and separate the leaves.
2. On a large serving plate, combine the leaves of the watercress and the spinach.
3. Cut the avocado in half, then remove the pit. Peel the skin off from each side.
4. Slice the avocados into thin strips. Set aside.
5. Prepare the dressing by combining avocado oil and lemon juice.
6. Arrange the avocado strips on top of the watercress and spinach.
7. Season with salt and pepper.
8. Drizzle with the dressing before serving.

Baked Salmon

Ingredients:
- 2 salmon fillets
- 6 cups of fresh spinach
- 2 tsp. coconut oil
- 1/4 tsp. garlic powder
- 1/4 tsp. turmeric
- 3 large cloves of garlic
- lemon juice
- salt
- pepper

Instructions:
1. Preheat the oven to 400°F.
2. Line a baking dish with parchment paper.
3. Marinate salmon fillets in lemon juice, coconut oil, garlic powder, turmeric, salt, and pepper.
4. Let it sit for a few minutes. This may also be done the night before to help the juices and flavor get into the salmon.
5. Once the oven is ready, bake the salmon for 15 minutes.
6. Cook some of the garlic in a pan with coconut oil.
7. Add spinach and cook until ready. Season with salt and pepper to taste.
8. Take salmon out of the oven and put spinach beside it.
9. Serve and enjoy.

Lemon Roasted Broccoli

Ingredients:
- 1-1/2 lb. broccoli florets
- 1/3 cup shredded Parmesan cheese
- 1/4 cup olive oil
- 2 tbsp. fresh basil, chopped
- 3 tsp. minced garlic
- 1/2 – 3/4 tsp. kosher salt
- 1/2 tsp. red chili flakes
- 1/2 lemon juice and zest

Instructions:
1. Preheat the oven to 425°F.
2. Line a baking sheet with parchment paper and spread the broccoli florets.
3. Season the broccoli with basil, olive oil, garlic, kosher salt, chili flakes, lemon zest, and lemon juice.
4. Sprinkle the top with parmesan cheese then put into the oven for 20-25 minutes or until the cheese has slightly melted.
5. Serve and enjoy while warm.

Flat Bread

Ingredients:
- 1 tbsp. ground psyllium husk powder
- 1/4 cup olive oil
- 1/2 cup coconut flour
- 1/3 cup grated parmesan cheese or mozzarella cheese
- 1 cup boiling water
- 1/2 tsp. sea salt
- 1/4 tsp. granulated garlic
- 1/2 tbsp. black peppercorns
- 1/2 tbsp. rosemary, dried

Instructions:
1. Whisk all the dry ingredients together in a mixing bowl.
2. Put olive oil and cheese in the mixture.
3. Pour in the hot water while stirring.
4. Don't stop stirring until the coconut flour and psyllium fiber have absorbed all of the water.
5. Flatten the dough onto parchment paper on a baking sheet, until it is 1/8-inch thin and even.
6. Bake for 20-25 minutes. Baking time will depend on the thickness of the dough.
7. When browned, transfer to a cooling rack, peel away the parchment paper, and allow the flatbread to cool.
8. Use a pizza cutter to cut the flatbread into squares for sandwiches.
9. Store any leftovers in the refrigerator.

Stuffed Chicken

Ingredients:
- 4 pcs. chicken breast filets, skinless and boneless
- 1/4 cup feta cheese, crumbled
- 1/4 cup artichoke hearts, finely chopped, drained, and marinated
- 2 tbsp. red peppers, finely chopped, drained, and roasted
- 2 tbsp. green onion, thinly sliced
- 2 tsp. fresh oregano, or 1/2 tsp. if using dried oregano
- 1 tsp. kosher salt
- 1/4 tsp. ground black pepper

Instructions:
1. Cut a pocket in each chicken breast using a sharp knife. Cut through the thickest portion horizontally without cutting through the opposite side.
2. Combine the feta, roasted peppers, artichoke hearts, oregano and green onions into a mixture.
3. Fill each pocket of the chicken breast with the mixture.
4. Close the opening of the pockets with a wooden toothpick.
5. Season the chicken breast with salt and pepper.
6. Preheat a non-stick large skillet on medium heat.
7. Coat it with cooking spray.
8. Fry the chicken for 10 to 12 minutes on each side, or until the internal temperature reaches at least 165°F.
9. Serve hot.

Grilled Lamb

Ingredients:
- 1-1/2 lb. baby spinach leaves
- 3 tbsp. dried oregano, chopped
- 1/4 cup lemon juice
- 1/4 cup olive oil
- 2 tbsp. ground cumin
- 1 tsp. crushed red pepper
- 1 tbsp. coarse sea salt
- 1 tbsp. squeezed juice from an orange
- 3 cloves garlic
- 2 yellow onions, chopped
- cooking spray

Instructions:
1. In a 2-gallon zip bag, put the lamb together with the lemon juice, oregano, cumin, and salt.
2. Close the bag and refrigerate overnight
3. Puree onions, garlic, some orange juice, and olive oil in a blender.
4. Transfer to a small bowl with a cover.
5. Chill overnight.
6. Mix sea salt, red pepper, and cumin in a small bowl
7. Remove refrigerated lamb and let it sit for 30 minutes.
8. Preheat the grill to medium.
9. Place lamb on the grill and coat with some cooking spray or oil.
10. Grill lamb for one and a half hours over medium heat.
11. Remove the lamb from the grill.
12. Serve hot.

Ground Beef Stroganoff

Ingredients:
- 1 lb. 80% lean ground beef
- 2 tbsp. butter
- 1 clove garlic, minced
- 10 oz. sliced mushrooms
- 1 tbsp. fresh parsley, chopped
- 1 tbsp. fresh lemon juice
- salt
- pepper
- 2 tbsp. water

Instructions:
1. Heat the large skillet over medium heat.
2. Put in the butter, letting it melt.
3. Add in the garlic and wait until it turns brown
4. Add beef and season with salt and pepper.
5. When the garlic turns brown, add the beef. Season with salt and pepper.
6. Drain some of the oil from the skillet.
7. Add the mushroom to the leftover oil and cook for 2 minutes. Add water.
8. Reduce the heat to low. Add the lemon juice.
9. Garnish with parsley and serve immediately.

Banana Bread

Ingredients:
- 1 cup olive oil mayonnaise
- 2 eggs
- 4 medium ripe bananas, mashed
- 2 tsp. vanilla extract
- 2 cups unbleached all-purpose flour
- 1 cup whole wheat flour
- 3/4 cup Brown Xylitol
- 2 tsp. baking soda
- 2 tsp. sea salt
- 2 tsp. cinnamon
- 1 tsp. baking powder
- Optional: flax, nuts, wheat germ, or whey protein

Instructions:
1. Preheat the oven to 350°F.
2. In a large mixing bowl, mix in banana, mayonnaise, eggs, and vanilla extract.
3. Combine the remaining dry ingredients in a different container.
4. Combine both mixtures by adding the dry one to the wet mixture.
5. Stir in the optional ingredients if desired.
6. Place the batter into a couple of loaf pans. Make sure to grease the pans first.
7. Place in the oven for about 45 to 50 minutes.
8. Let stand for 10 minutes. Remove from pan to finish cooling.
9. Serve and enjoy.

Healthy Green Smoothie

Ingredients:
- 1 cup fresh spinach
- 1/2 tsp. mint extract or to taste
- Optional: 1/4 tsp. peppermint liquid Stevia

Instructions:
1. Gather the ingredients.
2. Add them to a high-powered blender.
3. Turn on the blender.
4. Add them to the glass and freeze for 5 minutes.
5. Serve and enjoy.

Red Velvet Molten Lava Cake

Ingredients:
- 2 tbsp. coconut flour
- 1 tbsp. unsweetened cocoa powder
- 1 tbsp. ground flaxseed meal
- 1/2 tsp. baking powder
- 1/4 tsp. salt
- 1/4 cup 1% milk
- 1/4 tsp. vanilla extract
- 2 eggs
- 1 tsp. chocolate liquid stevia, or 1/2 cup of sugar-free sweetener
- 85% dark chocolate bars, broken into pieces
- 3 drops of red food coloring

Instructions:

1. Mix the coconut flour, cocoa powder, flaxseed, baking powder, and salt.
2. In a separate bowl, whisk the milk, eggs, vanilla extract, stevia, and food coloring together.
3. Pour the dry mixture into the wet mixture. Stir until combined.
4. Adjust food coloring to the redness you desire.
5. Spray oil on a couple of microwave-safe mugs or ramekins.
6. Pour batter into each container.
7. Insert chocolate pieces in the center of each batter.
8. Microwave one cake at a time for about one and a half minutes.
9. Serve and enjoy while warm.

Chicken Masala Crockpot Style

Ingredients:
- 6 boneless skinless chicken breasts, halved lengthwise
- 2 cloves of minced garlic
- 2 tbsp. extra virgin olive oil
- 1 tsp. salt
- 1 tsp. pepper
- 2 cups Marsala wine or chicken broth
- 1 cup of cold water
- 1/2 cup arrowroot powder
- 16 oz. sliced baby Portobello mushrooms
- 3 tbsp. fresh parsley, chopped

Instructions:
1. Grease the slow cooker. Add garlic and oil.
2. Season chicken with salt and pepper on each side and lay in the crockpot.
3. Pour wine over the chicken and cover the crockpot.
4. Cook on high for 3 hours.
5. Mix water with arrowroot and stir until absorbed.
6. Remove chicken from the crockpot and keep warm.
7. Stir in the arrowroot water mixture into the bottom of the crockpot. Add mushrooms.
8. Add back the chicken. Stir well to coat the chicken with sauce and mushrooms.
9. Cover and cook for an additional hour.
10. Serve with a sprinkle of chopped fresh parsley.

Balsamic-Glazed Chicken Thighs

Ingredients:
- 1 tsp. garlic powder
- 1 tsp. dried basil
- 1/2 tsp. salt
- 1/2 tsp. pepper
- 2 tsp. dehydrated onion
- 4 garlic cloves, minced
- 1 tbsp. extra-virgin olive oil
- 1/2 cup balsamic vinegar, divide equally
- 8 chicken thighs, boneless and skinless
- fresh chopped parsley, for garnish

Instructions:
1. In a small bowl, combine the onion, basil, garlic powder, salt, and pepper.
2. Spread the mixture over the chicken on both sides. Set aside.
3. Pour olive oil into the crockpot and add garlic.
4. Pour in half of the balsamic vinegar.
5. Place chicken on top.
6. Gently pour the remaining balsamic vinegar over the chicken.
7. Cover and cook on high for 3 hours.
8. Sprinkle fresh parsley on top to serve.

Zero Carb Buttery Noodles

Ingredients:
- 7 oz. shirataki noodles
- 2 tbsp. unsalted butter
- 1 tbsp. grated parmesan
- salt
- black pepper
- fresh basil or parsley

Instructions:
1. Drain and rinse the noodles in cold water.
2. Transfer them to a bowl, and cover them with boiling water for 5 minutes.
3. Drain again.
4. In a skillet, melt the butter over medium heat.
5. Add the noodles, and sprinkle in some salt.
6. Sauté for 3-4 minutes until the butter has been absorbed.
7. Add pepper to the task, and garnish with parmesan and basil or parsley.

Zero Carb Bread

Ingredients:
- 3 eggs
- 3 tbsp. cream cheese at room temperature
- 1/4 tsp. baking powder

Instructions:
1. Preheat the oven to 300°F.
2. Separate the yolk from the egg whites.
3. In one bowl, mix the egg yolks, cream cheese, and honey until smooth.
4. In a second bowl, add baking powder to the whites. Beat the whites with the hand mixer at high speed until they are fluffy.
5. Gently fold the egg yolk mixture into the egg white mixture.
6. Continue folding gently but swiftly to avoid melting the mixture. Make sure to not break the egg whites' fluffiness.
7. Spoon about 10-12 rounds of the mixture onto a lightly greased baking sheet.
8. Bake for 18-20 minutes on the middle rack.
9. Broil for a minute or a minute and a half, cooking the top until they become nice and golden brown.

Zero Carb Pizza Crust

Ingredients:
- 10 oz. canned chicken
- 1 oz. grated parmesan cheese
- 1 large egg

Instructions:
1. Drain the canned chicken thoroughly, getting as much moisture out as possible.
2. Spread chicken on a baking sheet lined with a silicone mat.
3. Bake at 350°F for 10 minutes to dry out the chicken.
4. Once it's done, remove it and place it in a mixing bowl. Increase the heat of the oven to 500°F.
5. Add cheese and egg to the bowl with chicken and mix.
6. Pour the mixture onto a baking sheet lined with a silicone mat.
7. Spread thinly. Place parchment paper on top and use a rolling pin to do so.
8. Optional: With a spatula, press in the edges of the crust to create a ridge, to keep any topping from falling off.
9. Bake the crust for 8-10 minutes at 500°F.
10. Remove the crust from the oven.
11. Add desired toppings and bake for another 6-10 minutes at 500°F. Toppings will dictate the final cook time.
12. Remove from the oven and allow to cool for a few minutes.
13. Serve and enjoy.

CONCLUSION

Carb cycling is an efficient and straightforward approach to dieting that can help women achieve their weight loss or maintenance goals. Carb cycling is a form of intermittent fasting that includes varying the number of carbohydrates consumed between high, low, and moderate levels while maintaining the same amounts of protein and fat. Women can discover the "sweet spot" that allows them to continue to eat their favorite foods while still making progress toward their ideal body composition by cycling the carbohydrates in their diet.

Carb cycling has been found in studies to increase metabolism, decrease fat reserves, and promote muscle building in addition to these benefits. Alterations in carbohydrate consumption help the body utilize calories differently and stimulate innovative meal planning with meals that are rich in nutrients. In addition, adhering to this sort of diet plan enables more flexibility than typically limited diets to do since women don't have to spend every day calculating calories or excluding whole food categories from their meals. This is because women don't have to follow traditional restricted diets.

Although the outcomes of a carb cycling diet may vary from one individual to the next, the majority of women report favorable outcomes such as increased levels of energy, improved digestion, enhanced quality of sleep, a reduction in cravings for unhealthy foods, an improved sense of control over their bodies and lives in general, and a more positive relationship with food.

You won't notice rapid results as you would with other types of fad diets; nonetheless, it is vital to keep in mind that altering your eating habits takes time. You will need the patience to get used to the new eating patterns and figure out how they work best for you.

However, if you are dedicated to and consistent with following the diet plan, as well as engaging in regular exercise routines that are associated with it, you should start seeing positive changes within a few weeks or months. Carb cycling, all things considered, provides many women who are searching for an easier way to control their weight without having to sacrifice their long-term health objectives with several beneficial options that they may choose from.

REFERENCES AND HELPFUL LINKS

Carb cycling for women: Sculpt your body while eating your fav foods. (2019, November 7). https://jcdfitness.com/2019/11/carb-cycling-for-women/.

DiLonardo, M. J. (n.d.). Carb cycling. WebMD. Retrieved March 25, 2023, from https://www.webmd.com/diet/carb-cycling-overview.

If keto and carb cycling had a baby it would be 'keto cycling'—Here's what to know about it. (2019, October 8). Women's Health. https://www.womenshealthmag.com/weight-loss/a19975595/carb-cycling-for-weight-loss/.

The beginner's guide to carb cycling. (n.d.). Shape. Retrieved March 25, 2023, from https://www.shape.com/healthy-eating/diet-tips/what-is-carb-cycling.

What is carb cycling and how does it work? (2022, August 3). Healthline. https://www.healthline.com/nutrition/carb-cycling-101.

Printed in Great Britain
by Amazon